SANDRA KNECHT

Guided Meditation Scripts

A Teaching Resource for Yoga Instructors, Life Coaches, Wellness Gurus and Healers

Contents

Preface

Feelings come and go
like clouds in a windy sky.

Conscious breathing
is my anchor.

Thich Nhat Hahn

1

Guided Meditation

"The mind is definitely something that can be transformed, and meditation is a means to transform it." – Dalai Lama

WHAT IS GUIDED MEDITATION?

Meditation is a mind-body technique that has been used for a very long time to increase tranquility and physical relaxation, enhance psychological equilibrium, cope with disease, and improve general health and well-being. The interplay between the brain, mind, body, and behavior are the main emphasis of mind-body activities.

In guided meditation, you will be led by a narrator to bring about a certain transformation in your life. Before embarking on an internal trip to accomplish a certain objective, you are instructed to unwind your body and mind, allowing you to reach an incredibly deep state of relaxation.

Guided meditation is especially beneficial for students who are having trouble focusing during their personal meditation practices. Oral instructions on proper posture for meditation, paying attention to the breath, body scanning procedures, and guided imagery or visualization are all examples of guided meditations. They can also involve chanting, saying aspirations out loud, or repeating mantras. They might even consist of particular motions or exercises done in a contemplative manner.

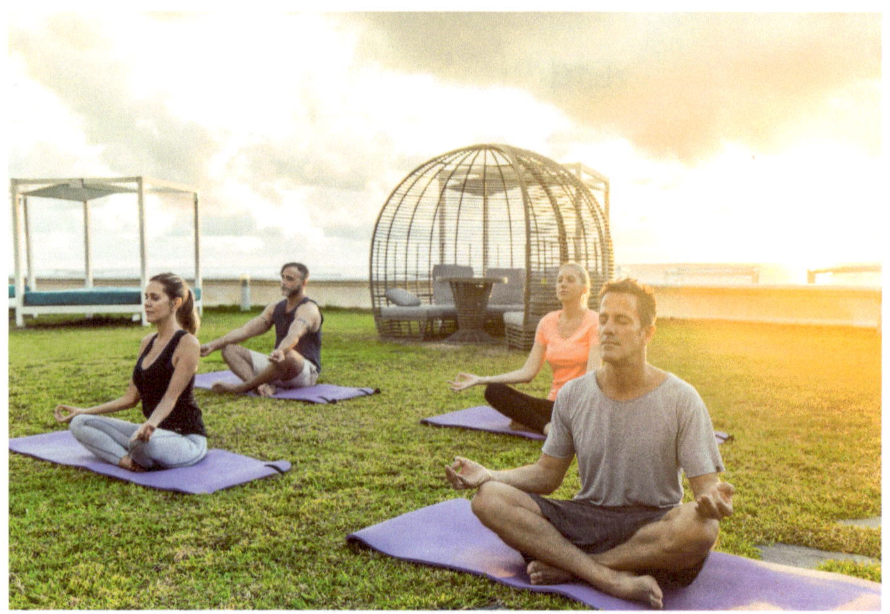

Photo by Jose Vazquez

2

Benefits of Guided Meditation

Meditation can improve your quality of life by providing numerous psychological and physical benefits. According to the science, meditation has the power to:

- Reduces Stress
  - Controls Anxiety
  - Promotes Emotional Health
  - Enhances Self Awareness
  - Lengthens Attention Span
  - May Reduce Age-Related Memory Loss
  - Can Generate Kindness
  - May Help Fight Addictions
  - Improves Sleep
  - Helps Control Pain
  - Can Decrease Blood Pressure
  - AND MUCH MORE!

People have long been aware of the many benefits of meditation. It is clear that meditation helps heal you mentally and physically, but when your meditation practice is over, the advantages don't end there. You will find that committing to a regular meditation practice will have profound effects on every aspect of your life.

How Often How Often Should You Meditate and for How Long?

It's up to you. If possible, meditate daily for at least 10 minutes. When we develop a regular meditation practice, we notice the most benefits. With consistency, mindfulness skills grow stronger and integrating mindfulness practices into daily life becomes more intuitive. That's when the real transformation begins. Try starting to mediate once a day for at least 10 minutes and work your way up from there.

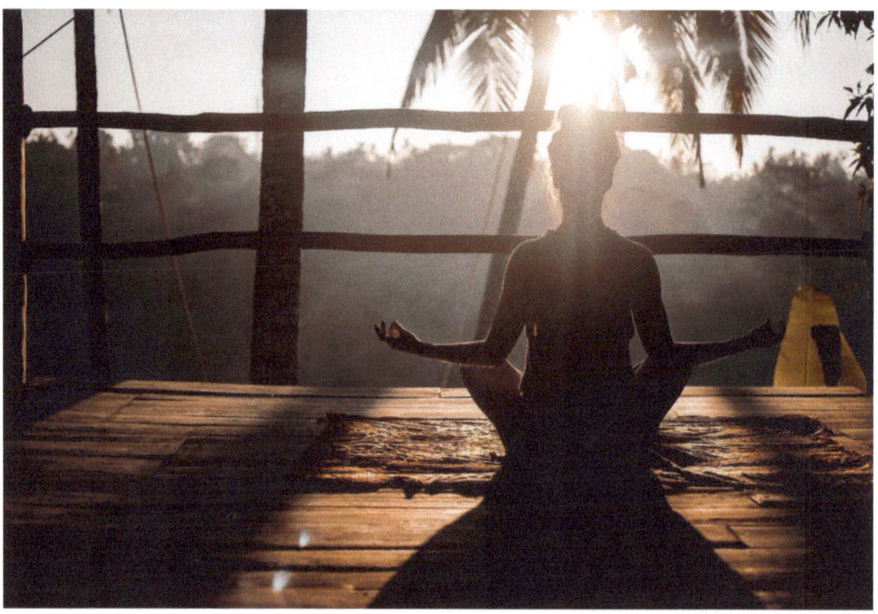

Photo by Jared Rice

3

Leading Guided Meditations

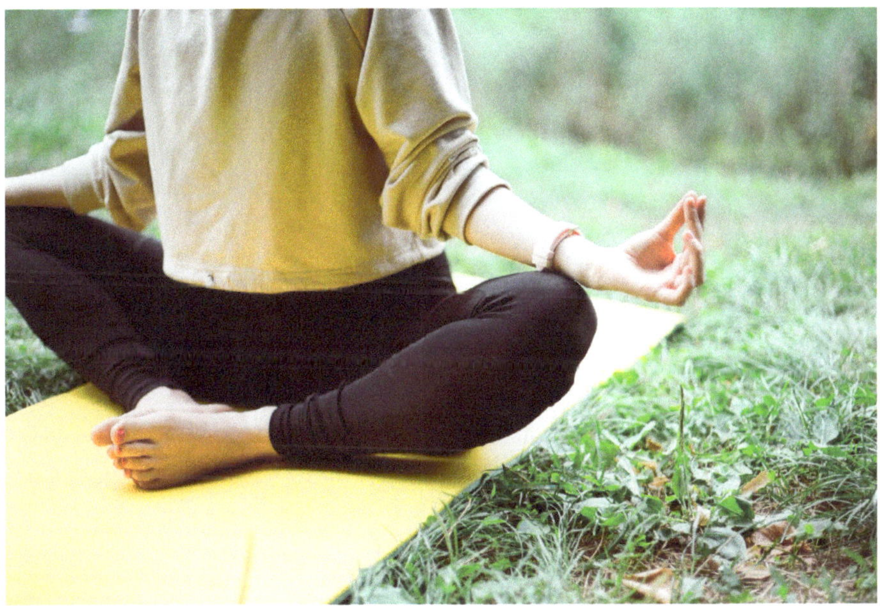

The role of the teacher is to lead their participants through an inner experience with a specific goal. That goal could be as simple as relaxing their body and mind or as complex as a guided journey that includes visualization techniques and thought-provoking questions throughout the meditation experience. Steps to comfortably introduce students to meditation as a coping strategy for stress and to effectively guide them through a meditation session, follow these steps:

STEP 1

Begin with a Topic & Discussion Beginning a guided meditation with a brief discussion is important so that you can capture the focus and attention of your students/clients. People live highly stimulated & distracted lives today. A brief discussion around a quote captures their attention and allows them to transition from their previous activities to the meditation experience. They will be able to shift into an introspective mind-state. They will need to access this to have an insightful and meaningful meditation experience.

STEP 2

Get Everyone Comfortable & Prepare the Room Having a comfortable student is essential while leading a guided meditation. It is your job as the teacher to ensure that the space is properly set up and protected from unexpected interruptions. Here are some examples of things you'll want to consider while preparing your participants & the room for a guided meditation: • Will they be seated or lying down? (Either is OK, but try having them lie down if possible) • Consider bringing eye covers to help people maintain their inward focus • Play gentle meditation music if possible to fill the space between your words

  • Make sure everyone's phones are off or on airplane mode to avoid interruptions • Lock or place a sign on the door to avoid any unexpected visitors during your meditation • Once you've decided on all these things and set the room up accordingly, have everyone take their seats or lie down, turn the lights down or off, and move on to the next step.

STEP 3

Start the Meditation with a Progressive Relaxation Once everyone is comfortable, your music is playing and you are in a comfortable position to begin, you are ready to start the meditation. The beginning is important because this is where your participants will shift into a meditative state. Your guidance is very important here for setting the correct pace of breathing that will result in the meditative state your audience desires. In the beginning, it's up to you to guide them on the correct rhythm of inhalation & exhalation. Avoid rushing through this critical aspect. Count SILENTLY to yourself. For example, if it suits your teaching style you could try 5 seconds on the inhalation, 2 seconds at the top of the breath, 4 seconds on the exhalation, and 2 seconds at the bottom of the breath. While you are letting them settle into this experience, offer reminders to release tension in the area around their eyes, their jaws, and in their shoulders. This is the most important part of the meditation, so allow at least 6 minutes for this step. Don't rush the pace of their breathing & engage in the meditation as you are guiding them with the use of the scripts in this book. This will help you stay in rhythm with your participants' cycles of breath.

STEP FOUR

Allow Time for Silent Reflection The most valuable part of a guided meditation is not when you are talking; it's when you are silent. Throughout your guidance of the meditation, let your audience know that your voice will be silent for a time, and give them as much time as you can allow to listen from within. Prepare your students for insight provoking moments of reflection by asking your group to find peace and comfort in your periodic silences.

STEP FIVE

Slowly, Bring People Back to Your Voice After a sufficient amount of silent time has passed, gently reintroduce your voice by saying something like, "And slowly, coming back to the sound of my voice." Then, have your participants begin to wiggle their toes and fingers and bring their attention back into their bodies. Before moving on to the final step, make sure to ask your participants to take something with them from the experience. This can be a realization or a simple recognition of a feeling. Prompting a takeaway in this manner is important to help your audience remember the experience as they go forward and bring something of value with them. STEP 6: Bring Your Audience to Waking Consciousness Finally, ask your participants to open their eyes. You may end this part in any way that you see fit for the given situation. However, I suggest that you end by suggesting a conscious action to acknowledge the experience & solidify any insights into their memory. If possible, have them write for a few minutes in a journal, about anything. If that's not possible, simply asking everyone to stay off their phones for at least 10 minutes will suffice (Varnum, Hunter One Soul Stream, 2019). Preparation: • Adapt, adjust and rehearse guided meditation yourself so you will be comfortable slowing down and pacing. • Identify key words to pre-teach • Experiment with calming lighting in the room.

TIPS FOR LEADING A MEDITATION

Guiding others in meditation may feel daunting or nerve wracking at first, but it is just like taking a client through any other exercise. You've got this!

Here are a few tips for leading guided meditation sessions:

Use a notebook, a word processor, or free tools like Canva to outline your entire teaching sessions. Create "workbooks" and "handouts" for your students with key terms, "homework" assignments, short spiritual reading assignments etc. Handing out visual aids and reading material shows your level of compassion and preparation. Your clients will appreciate how deeply dedicated you are to supporting them throughout their healing journeys.

Familiarize yourself with meditation postures. It is important to keep the spine straight, the hands supported, and the body relaxed. Incorporate yin yoga poses into your guided meditation sessions.

Buy a stopwatch. It is best not to use the stopwatch on your phone because you want to minimize distractions and reduce the risk of any unwanted interruptions.

Ensure you know the practice yourself well before guiding others. Your degree of familiarity with the practice will become evident through the confidence that shines through more and more as you guide sessions more frequently. It is SO IMPORTANT to intentionally put yourself in a student mindset outside of your own classes. As a teacher, swallow your pride and attend other teachers' classes with a completely open mind and a jovial spirit. Remain curious about your craft and hungry for new experiences that could expand on your own expertise.

Pace your delivery of meditation scripts with a gentle and patient spirit. When in doubt, slow your pace down. Slow delivery is always better than fast delivery when it comes to meditation. Remember that your clients are looking forward to relaxing, so there is no need to rush. Get comfortable with pauses. The silence is an important part of a meditation session. Practice finding comfort in these moments.

Attend classes. This will give you the opportunity to continuously expand your teaching "toolbox". Keep an open heart and try to get as much as you can out of every class you attend. Remember, you can learn something from everyone.

Keep your tone of voice calm and measured. Some people are naturally endowed with a soothing voice, others can practice by recording themselves first and spending a lot of time learning from other teachers.

Write out all of your guided meditation scripts before you use them in class. Consider recording your guided meditations before guiding large groups. As soon as you feel comfortable ditching the script, go ahead and do so. I don't recommend memorizing scripts and just regurgitating them, but I do recommend taking this book out and simply reading the scripts in a slowly paced, calming and reassuring tone SEVERAL TIMES before you attempt to set the book down and start winging it. Once you feel comfortable and confident with a particular meditation and you feel like you've altered the phrasing to suit your natural speech patterns, go ahead and let your uniqueness shine!

If you are new to guiding large groups, start out with candle meditations. Face your students against the wall and pass out tea lights. Have your students light the tea lights in front of them and instruct them to breathe and focus on the candle flame during the meditation. This strategy will take some of the pressure and anxiety away from you because you are able to redirect the visual focus of your students. Just as your students are on a mindfulness journey, so are you. Remember to be patient and kind with yourself as well. You cannot pour from an empty cup!

4

Preparing the Space

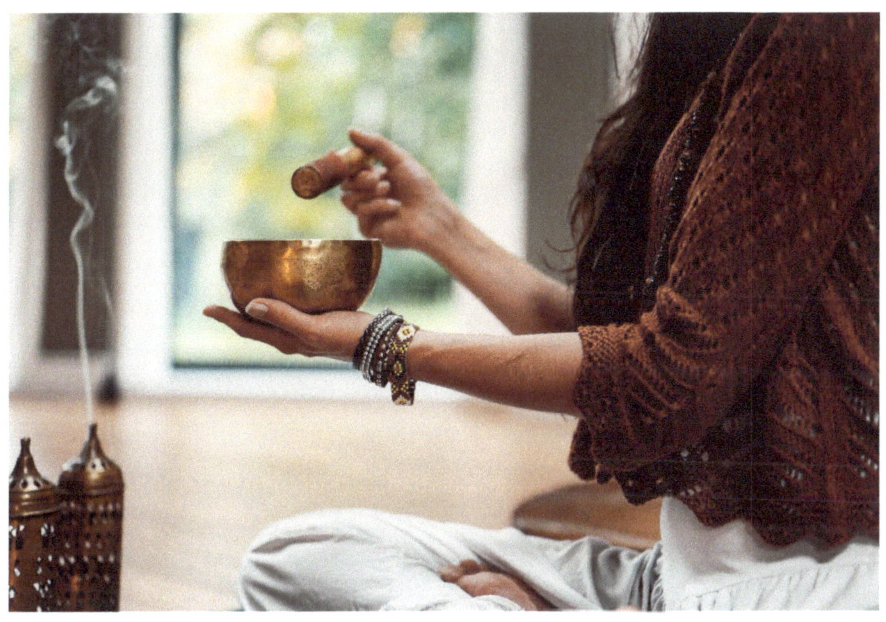

BEFORE EACH SESSION:

Allow everyone to get seated, attentive and comfortable. Allow people to chat for a few minutes among themselves. *This helps everyone ground themselves in unfamiliar environments and social groups.*

Pass around some props (may include, not limited to):

- blankets
- cushions
- workbooks, worksheets, handouts, books
- tea lights, candles
- essential oils
- eye masks
- straps
- blocks

Take several minutes to help students fold blankets, adjust bolsters, blocks, and just help them get comfortable. Dim the lights if you haven't already. Incorporate soothing stimuli like gentle music or therapeutic nature sounds playing through a reliable speaker. Set the thermostat at 70-72 degrees for a meditation session. Avoid a space that is too cold or too warm. Students will be using blankets and pillows while they are meditating, so anything warmer than 72 may be uncomfortable.

5

Meditation and The Breath

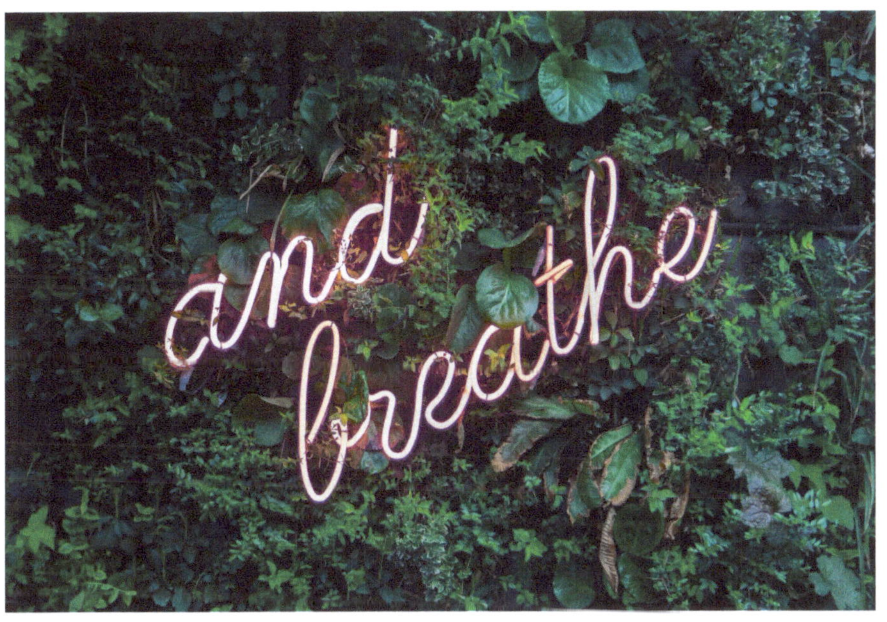

Breath Awareness

Introducing your students to essential breathing techniques

Those who meditate often strive to cultivate a conscious breath in their practice. Understanding breathing techniques will help you deepen your practice and increase the connection between mind and body. The foundation of any meditation practice is the breath. In yoga and many forms of meditation, proper breathing techniques are referred to as pranayama. The Sanskrit term "prana" means life force energy, and "ayama" means to free or extend. Therefore pranayama is the control of our life force energy through conscious regulation of our breath. Before guiding your students through the following meditations, I recommend educating them on the following: The Natural Breath Although it's not technically a breathing technique because it's not controlling the breath, the natural breath is the basis for your meditation practice. The natural breath is not manipulated in any way. For example, when lying in meditation at the end of the practice, the breath is naturally flowing, as we have surrendered and released into the practice. However, many of us have abandoned our natural breath, as stress, tension, and pain all affect how we breathe. Over time we habituate an unhealthy breathing pattern, originating from the upper chest, rather than the abdomen. When our breath resides in the upper chest it's shallow, making it difficult for enough oxygen to enter. Take time throughout your meditation practice, especially at the beginning to become aware of your natural breath at that moment. The Full Yogic Breath When practicing the full yogic breath we breathe into three sectors of the torso one at a time, then release the breath one sector at a time. First inhale into the belly, extending outward. Pause. Then inhale into the mid chest as the ribs expand to the front, back and sides. Pause. Then inhale into the upper chest, the area just under your collar bones. Progressively filling up from bottom to top, creating expansion in all directions. Then gradually release the breath without forcing it out.

6

Pranayama Fact Sheet

Instructor Resource: Pranayama Fact Sheet

1. Yogic Breath Control

Yoga and the breath are intricately connected. Yogi's strive to cultivate a conscious breath in their practice. Understanding the yogic breath will help you deepen your practice and increase the connection between mind and body. The foundation of any yoga practice is the breath. The Sanskrit term "prana" means life force energy, and "ayama" means to free or extend. Therefore pranayama is the control of our life force energy through conscious regulation of our breath.

2. The Natural Breath

Although it's not technically a pranayama practice because it's not controlling the breath, the natural breath is the basis for your pranayama practice. The natural breath is not manipulated in any way . For example, when lying in meditation at the end of a yoga practice the breath is naturally flowing, as we surrender and release into the pose. However, many of us have abandoned our natural breath, as stress, tension, and pain all affect how we breathe. Over time we habituate an unhealthy breathing pattern, originating from the upper chest, rather than the abdomen. When our breath resides in the upper chest it's shallow, making it difficult for enough oxygen to enter. Take time throughout your yoga practice, especially at the beginning to become aware of your natural breath at that moment.

3. The Full Yogic Breath

When practicing the full yogic breath we breathe into three sectors of the torso one at a time, then release the breath one sector at a time. First inhale into the belly, extending outward. Pause. Then inhale into the mid chest as the ribs expand to the front, back and sides. Pause. Then inhale into the upper chest, the area just under your collar bones. Progressively filling up from bottom to top, creating expansion in all directions. Then gradually release the breath without forcing it out.

4. Ujjayi Breath (pronounced oo-jye)

The ujjayi breath is done through the nostrils with the lips closed. The breath is even and steady. There is a slight contraction at the back of the throat which will make a subtle hissing sound. Basically it's like you're trying to fog up a mirror but with the mouth closed. The inhalation and exhalation should be slightly audible. This breath is often done during a yoga practice, pairing inhalation and exhalation with the movements in and out of poses. It builds heat in the body and connects you to the flow of the breath. According to BKS Iyengar this is also good for those suffering from low blood pressure, asthma, and depression, as it invigorates the nervous system. You may also hear Ujjayi Breath referred to as Oceanic Breath.

Keep in Mind: *Only four types of basic yogic breathing exercises are introduced here. There are many more pranayama exercises that you can research and incorporate into your meditation practice.*

7

Breath Awareness Meditation Script

Script and Guidance Tips:

- *Prepare the space for your students. Adjust the lighting, music, etc to create a calming and space environment*
- *Engage your students with a brief story, quote, or topic related to the following meditation to help shift their focus onto the practice*
- *On average, you should pause for 3 seconds between each line of the script*

—BEGIN READING HERE—

"Come to a comfortable position lying on your back.

Take a moment to get comfortable here and begin to focus on the natural rhythm of your breath.

Inhale slowly and smoothly allowing the breath to travel deeply into the low belly.

Pause and exhale slowly and smoothly releasing the breath from the body

through your nostrils or out of your mouth."

- *Pause here for a few minutes in silence and let your students enter into a more relaxed and introspective space. Remind your students that your voice will be absent periodically throughout the practice. This is intentional - the silence allows them to turn their focus inward on their own journey through the practice.*
- *Remember to insert as many additional pauses as you need to. Your goal is to sound authentic and natural.*

"Now take a moment to make any last minute adjustments here so that your body can remain as comfortable and still as possible throughout this practice.

Feel the breath flowing in and flowing out.

Soften your face and jaw to allow the breath to flow smoothly in and smoothly out.

Soften the eyes and relax the shoulders.

Let your entire body feel relaxed and heavy.

Weighted and secure.

And now, slowly come back to the sound of my voice.

Continue to breathe and let any distracting thoughts float away from you.

Breathe in through your nose and out through your nose or mouth.

Allow your breath to find its own natural rhythm.

Bring your full attention to the sensations of each inhale as the air enters your nostrils, travels throughout your lungs and causes your belly to expand.

Take the time to notice each exhale as your belly contracts and air moves up through the lungs back up and exits through your nose or mouth.

Invite your full attention to flow with your breath and notice all of the associated sensations in every area of your body.

Notice how the inhale is different from the exhale. You may experience the air as cool as it enters your nose and warm as you exhale.

Turn inward and begin to let go of the distractions around you.

Begin to let go of the noises around you,

And if they become a distraction at any point, briefly take note them and then bring your attention back to your breath.

Don't worry about trying to change anything about your breathing. Don't try to control it.

Observe and accept your experience in this moment without judgment, feeling gratitude for each inhale and exhale.

If your mind wanders to thoughts, plans or problems, simply notice your mind wandering.

Observe the thought as it enters your awareness as neutrally as possible.

Then let it go as if it were a fluffy cloud simply floating across the sky above you.

In your minds eye, place each thought that arises on a cloud and watch as it floats out of your view.

Then bring your attention back to your breath.

Always come back to the breath.

Your inhales and exhales are meant to function as the anchors that you may return to over and over again when you become distracted by intrusive thoughts or emotions.

Notice when your mind wanders and

Noticing is the richest part of learning. Observe the types of thoughts that tend to hook and distract you. With this knowledge you can strengthen your ability to detach from thoughts and mindfully focus your awareness back on the qualities of your breath.

Practice coming home to your body and breath with full attention.

Watch the gentle rise of your stomach on the in-breath and the relaxing, letting go on the out-breath.

Allow yourself to be completely with your breath as it flows in and out.

You might become distracted by pain or discomfort in the body or twitching or itching sensations that draw your attention away from the breath.

You may also notice feelings.

Perhaps sadness or happiness, frustration or contentment.

Acknowledge whatever comes up including thoughts or stories about your experience.

Simply notice where your mind went without judging it, pushing it away, clinging to it or wishing it were different.

Breathe in.

Breathe out.

And let it all go.

Refocus your mind and guide your attention back to your breath.

Breathe in and breathe out.

Follow the air all the way in

and all the way out.

Mindful and calm. Peaceful and still.

Stay present with this.

Mindful and calm. Peaceful and still.

Remain here for a few breaths.

Feeling mindful and calm.

Peaceful

and still.

Slowly… allow your attention to expand.

Begin wiggle your fingers and toes.

Take a few gentle breaths in and out.

Now, open your eyes slowly and give yourself a few moments to readjust to your physical surroundings.

When you are ready, roll on to your right side and push yourself back up to a seated position.

Before you leave class today, don't forget to thank yourself

for showing up on your mat today to nurture your mind, body, and spirit.

And thank you all so much for sharing this practice with me today.

Namaste.

8

Deep Breathing Meditation Script

Script and Guidance Tips:

- *Prepare the space for your students. Adjust the lighting, music, etc to create a calming and space environment*
- *Engage your students with a brief story, quote, or topic related to the following meditation to help shift their focus onto the practice*
- *On average, you should pause for 3 seconds between each line of the script*

—BEGIN READING HERE—

"Come to a comfortable position lying on your back.

Take a moment to get comfortable here and begin to focus on the natural rhythm of your breath.

Inhale slowly and smoothly allowing the breath to travel deeply into the low belly.

Pause and exhale slowly and smoothly releasing the breath from the body

through your nostrils or out of your mouth."

- ***Pause here for a few minutes in silence and let your students enter into a more relaxed and introspective space. Remind your students that your voice will be absent periodically throughout the practice. This is intentional - the silence allows them to turn their focus inward on their own journey through the practice.***
- ***Remember to insert as many additional pauses as you need to. Your goal is to sound authentic and natural.***

"Now take a moment to make any last minute adjustments here so that your body can remain as comfortable and still as possible throughout this practice.

Feel the breath flowing in and flowing out.

Soften your face and jaw to allow the breath to flow smoothly in and smoothly out.

Soften the eyes and relax the shoulders.

Let your entire body feel relaxed and heavy.

Weighted and secure.

And now, slowly come back to the sound of my voice.

Continue to breathe naturally and let any distracting thoughts float away from you.

Relax your body by releasing any areas of tension.

Adjust your upper body by pulling your shoulder blades down your back.

Tuck your chin toward your chest to lengthen the back of your neck.

Bring your feet as wide as your mat and let them flop open like a book.

Let your arms gently fall alongside your body, palms facing up.

If you'd like to take some pressure off your lower back, you can place a folded blanket or bolster under your knees.

You may also want to cover yourself with a blanket for warmth or anxiety relief.

[Give everyone ample time to situate themselves comfortably with blankets and props]

Now, close your eyes and let's settle in to stillness.

Close your eyes and take these first few moments to connect with your breath.

Observe your natural breath.

Feel the cool air as it enters your body and observe the depth and quality of your breath right now without any judgment.

Continue to connect with your breath and give yourself permission to completely relax now….

Allow your body to become heavy as if its sinking into the floor beneath you.

Let's begin to deepen the breath now.

We are going to breathe in for four counts, pause after our inhale for three counts, and then exhale for six counts.

Okay, deeeep breath in.
   Feel your belly rise and your rib cage expanding for
   One…. Two….. Three…… Four
   Now hold for
   One….. Two…..Three
   Aaaand exhale slowly
   One…. Two….. Three…. Four…. Five…. Six

And now, let's do that again.

Deeeeep breath in.
   Inhaling for
   One….Two….Three….Four….
   Holding for
   One…Two…Three..
   and Exhaling
   One…Two…Three…Four…Five…and Six

One more time.

Feel your belly rise and your rib cage expanding
   One…. Two….. Three…… Four
   Hold for
   One….. Two…..Three
   Aaand exhale
   One…. Two….. Three…. Four…. Five…and Six

Return to your natural breath and take a moment to visualize all of the fresh and revitalizing oxygen that is currently traveling throughout your entire body.

Allow your body to become very heavy, trusting that it is fully supported by the ground beneath you.

Part your lips slightly and relax your jaw.

Now, place your right hand on your belly and your left hand on your chest.

With the next inhalation, think of intentionally sending the air towards the navel by letting your abdomen expand and rise freely.

Feel the right hand rising while the left hand remains almost still on top of the chest.

Feel the right hand coming down as you exhale while keeping the abdomen relaxed.

Continue to repeat this for a few minutes without straining the abdomen. Just allow it to expand and relax freely.

After some repetitions, return to your natural breathing and allow yourself to rest quietly for a few moments.

Without changing your position, go ahead and shift your attention to your rib cage.

With the next inhalation, think of intentionally sending the air towards your rib cage instead of the abdomen.

Let your chest expand and rise freely, allowing your left hand to move up and down as you keep breathing.

Take another deep breath and shift your focus and your breath to your abdomen.

Inhale deeply and allow your belly to rise.

Pause for a moment then exhale slowly, allowing your belly to sink back down.

Your right hand should remain almost still.

Continue to this breathing pattern for the next few minutes on your own.

[silence for 60 seconds]

After some repetitions, return to your natural breathing and let's all rest quietly for a few moments now.

[silence for 120 seconds]

With your next inhalation,you are going to repeat a thoracic breathing pattern.

When the rib cage is completely expanded, inhale a bit more thinking of allowing the air to fill the upper section of your lungs at the base of your neck.

Feel the shoulders and collar bone rise up gently to find some space for the extra air to come in.

Exhale slowly letting the collarbone and shoulders drop first and then continue to relax the rib cage.

Continue to breathe like this for the next few minutes.

Acknowledge your thoughts briefly and then allow them to simply…. float away

Remember that you can always revisit any of these thoughts or feelings later….

but right now… if they are not serving you ……just let them drift off..

Deepen your inhales and exhales and do your best to maintain a consistent and silky smooth flow of breath

Continue to breathe and turn your attention inward now.

Tune into your body and accept all of the sensations you are experiencing with loving kindness.

Breathe naturally and allow yourself to rest in stillness and silence for the next few minutes.

[silence for 3-5 minutes]
  [bell/gong]

Begin to wiggle your fingers and toes.

Keeping your eyes closed, roll over onto your right side and push yourself up into a comfortable seated position.

On your next inhale, raise both of your arms up over your head and bring the palms of your hands together.

Keep your palms pressed together, and on your next inhale exhale, lower your hands down to a prayer position at heart center.

Gently flutter your eyes back open now and give yourself a little bow to honor yourself for taking this time for you.

Thank you guys so much for practicing with me today.

Namaste.

9

Visualization Meditation Script

Script and Guidance Tips:

- *Prepare the space for your students. Adjust the lighting, music, etc to create a calming and space environment*
- *Engage your students with a brief story, quote, or topic related to the following meditation to help shift their focus onto the practice*
- *On average, you should pause for 3 seconds between each line of the script*

—BEGIN READING HERE—

"Come to a comfortable position lying on your back.

Take a moment to get comfortable here and begin to focus on the natural rhythm of your breath.

Inhale slowly and smoothly allowing the breath to travel deeply into the low belly.

Pause and exhale slowly and smoothly releasing the breath from the body

through your nostrils or out of your mouth."

- *Pause here for a few minutes in silence and let your students enter into a more relaxed and introspective space. Remind your students that your voice will be absent periodically throughout the practice. This is intentional - the silence allows them to turn their focus inward on their own journey through the practice.*
- *Remember to insert as many additional pauses as you need to. Your goal is to sound authentic and natural.*

"Now take a moment to make any last minute adjustments here so that your body can remain as comfortable and still as possible throughout this practice.

Feel the breath flowing in and flowing out.

Soften your face and jaw to allow the breath to flow smoothly in and smoothly out.

Soften the eyes and relax the shoulders.

Let your entire body feel relaxed and heavy.

Weighted and secure.

And now, slowly come back to the sound of my voice.

Continue to breathe and let any distracting thoughts float away from you.

Relax your body by releasing any areas of tension.

Allow your arms to go limp... then your legs.... Feel your arms and legs becoming loose and relaxed...

Now relax your neck and back by relaxing your spine....

release the hold of your muscles all the way from your head, down your neck....along each vertebra to the tip of your spine...

Breathe deeply into your diaphragm, drawing air fully into your lungs.... and release the air with a whooshing sound....

Breathe in again, slowly.... pause for a moment.... and breathe out.....

Draw a deep breath in.... and out....

Become more and more relaxed with each breath....

Feel your body giving up tension....

You are becoming relaxed.... and calm.... peaceful....

Feel a wave of relaxation flow from the soles of your feet, to your ankles, lower legs, hips, pelvic area, abdomen, chest, back, hands, lower arms, elbows, upper arms, shoulders, neck, back of your head, face, and the top of your head....

Allow your entire body to rest heavily on the surface below you...

Now that your body is fully relaxed..Imagine you are walking toward the ocean.... ..through a beautiful, tropical forest....

You can hear the waves up ahead....

you can smell the ocean spray…and the air is warm against your skin.….

You feel a pleasant, cool breeze blowing through the trees.….

You walk along a path.….coming closer to the sea.….

As you come to the edge of the trees, you see the brilliant aqua color of the ocean ahead.….

You walk out of the forest and onto a long stretch of white sand.….

the sand is very fine and it glimmers in the sunlight.….

imagine yourself taking off your shoes, and walking through the hot, white sand toward the water.….

You hear the waves crashing to the shore.…. You smell the clean salt water…

You gaze again toward the water.…. it is a bright blue-green.….

The waves are washing up onto the sand.….. and receding back toward the ocean.…. washing up.….

and flowing back down.…..

Take a moment to enjoy the ever-repeating rhythm of the waves…

Imagine yourself walking toward the water.…. over the fine, hot sand.….

As you approach the water, you can feel the mist from the ocean on your skin.

You walk closer to the waves, and feel the sand becoming wet and firm.….

A wave washes over the sand toward you…. and touches your toes before receding…

As you step forward, more waves wash over your feet…

The cool water on your skin is providing you some relief from the heat now….

Walk further into the clear, clean water….

You look down and you can see the white sand under the water….you even notice a few small fishes swimming around nearby

The water is a pleasant, relaxing temperature…. providing relief from the hot sun…

You wade further into the water ….

You start to swim around now…. .and you're truly enjoying everything little thing about this moment.

You feel so calm and refreshed… and you stay in the water for awhile

When you finally get out of the water and onto the beach… you decide to stroll along the beach at the water's edge…. free of worries… no stress… calm….. enjoying this holiday….

Up ahead is a comfortable lounge chair and towel waiting, just for you…

You lie down in the chair and you're enjoying the sun on your skin….

the breeze…. the waves…..

You feel peaceful and relaxed….

All your stress is melting away….

When you are ready to return from your vacation, do so slowly….

Bring yourself back to your usual level of alertness and awareness….

But keep this feeling of calm and relaxation with you for the rest of your day….

Take a deep breath in. And breathe out.

And another deep breath in and let it go.

Open your eyes slowly and give yourself a few moments to readjust to your physical surroundings.

When you are ready, roll on to your right side and push yourself back up to a seated position.

Before you leave class today, don't forget to thank yourself

for showing up on your mat today to nurture your mind, body, and spirit.

And thank you all so much for sharing this practice with me today.

Namaste.

10

Mindfulness Meditation Script

Script and Guidance Tips:

- *Prepare the space for your students. Adjust the lighting, music, etc to create a calming and space environment*
- *Engage your students with a brief story, quote, or topic related to the following meditation to help shift their focus onto the practice*
- *On average, you should pause for 3 seconds between each line of the script*

—BEGIN READING HERE—

"Come to a comfortable position lying on your back.

Take a moment to get comfortable here and begin to focus on the natural rhythm of your breath.

Inhale slowly and smoothly allowing the breath to travel deeply into the low belly.

Pause and exhale slowly and smoothly releasing the breath from the body

through your nostrils or out of your mouth."

- *Pause here for a few minutes in silence and let your students enter into a more relaxed and introspective space. Remind your students that your voice will be absent periodically throughout the practice. This is intentional - the silence allows them to turn their focus inward on their own journey through the practice.*
- *Remember to insert as many additional pauses as you need to. Your goal is to sound authentic and natural.*

"Now take a moment to make any last minute adjustments here so that your body can remain as comfortable and still as possible throughout this practice.

Feel the breath flowing in and flowing out.

Soften your face and jaw to allow the breath to flow smoothly in and smoothly out.

Soften the eyes and relax the shoulders.

Let your entire body feel relaxed and heavy.

Weighted and secure.

And now, slowly come back to the sound of my voice.

Continue to breathe and let any distracting thoughts float away from you.

Now, bring your attention to your feet.

Imagine that your feet have grown deep roots into the earth beneath you.

Feel your strong foundation and deep connection to the earth.
As your foundation becomes stronger and your body relaxes further

Feel unwanted energy being pulled down from your head to your feet and back into the earth.

If your mind begins to wander, bring your focus back to the flow of your breath.

From here bring move your attention from your feet to your calves. Scanning from your toes up to your thighs.

Notice what you notice.

Sensations. Images.

Thoughts. Feelings.

Whatever you experience is perfect in this moment.

If you don't notice anything, that is also perfect.

Just be with the lower half of your body, visualizing the breath traveling there and nourishing

Shift your attention to the center of your belly.

Your gut provides valuable information to you on a daily basis.

Information that flows into your brain, whether you are aware of it or not.

Placing your hand on your belly, notice what you notice.

If anything arises a sensation, an image, a voice… just be with it.

Again, there is nothing your need to do right now.

There is no where you need to go.

Give yourself permission to release the tension from your body and mind. You do not have to carry the heaviness with you anymore. It was never yours to carry.

Rest comfortably and return to the breath.

Visualize it traveling to all the areas of your body that require a little extra attention.

Envision the oxygen swirling around any painful or tense spots, nourishing them deeply.

Giving your belly a gentle embrace, shift your focus to the core of your heart.

If it helps, move your hand over your heart.

Allowing your heart to beat in its natural rhythm, you might again find an image or sensation arise.

Listen within.

Listen deeply.

Be with whatever arises. And if your mind wanders, bring your attention back to the flow of your breath.

Now, shift your focus to the crown of your head as you open your focus to the spaciousness of the sky above.

A sky that is unlimited is potential and endless in possibilities.

Just like you.

Breathe deeply and exhale slowly and evenly.

Absorb the peaceful energy surrounding you in this space.

And now, as our meditation draws to a close,

gently open your eyes and reconnect with your surroundings.

Rise back up to seated when you feel ready to do so.

Thank you all for coming to class and sharing this experience with me today.

Namaste.

11

Deep Healing Meditation Script

Script and Guidance Tips:

- ***Prepare the space for your students. Adjust the lighting, music, etc to create a calming and space environment***
- ***Engage your students with a brief story, quote, or topic related to the following meditation to help shift their focus onto the practice***
- ***On average, you should pause for 3 seconds between each line of the script***

—BEGIN READING HERE—

"Come to a comfortable position lying on your back.

Take a moment to get comfortable here and begin to focus on the natural rhythm of your breath.

Inhale slowly and smoothly allowing the breath to travel deeply into the low belly.

Pause and exhale slowly and smoothly releasing the breath from the body

through your nostrils or out of your mouth."

- *Pause here for a few minutes in silence and let your students enter into a more relaxed and introspective space. Remind your students that your voice will be absent periodically throughout the practice. This is intentional - the silence allows them to turn their focus inward on their own journey through the practice.*
- *Remember to insert as many additional pauses as you need to. Your goal is to sound authentic and natural.*

"Now take a moment to make any last minute adjustments here so that your body can remain as comfortable and still as possible throughout this practice.

Feel the breath flowing in and flowing out.

Soften your face and jaw to allow the breath to flow smoothly in and smoothly out.

Soften the eyes and relax the shoulders.

Let your entire body feel relaxed and heavy.

Weighted and secure.

And now, slowly come back to the sound of my voice.

Continue to breathe and let any distracting thoughts float away from you.

Feel the breath as it enters with a cool feeling and then warming as it gently travels down into the lungs.

Fill the lungs with a deep inhale, bringing in energy and vitality.

As you exhale, feel the body releasing toxins, stress and negativity.

Stay with this breath, focusing on the feeling of deep peace for several deep inhalations and exhalations….

Feel the energy that is in the body.

Become aware of the warmth and tingling of every tiny cell that composes your entire being.

Feel the energy that surrounds you right now.

Feel the energy in every part of nature and in every living thing…..and bring all of that energy together and feel them as one.

Visualize all of that energy as a gigantic orb of bright white light - a divine healing light force.

Summon the shining orb of bright white light to hover directly over the crown of the head now.

Feel it starting to travel down into your body from the top of your head,

slowly moving down through your face and neck,

traveling down into the shoulders,

all the way down into the arms, and through each and every fingertip.

Feel the healing energy and light moving down into your chest, throughout the abdomen and all the way down to your hips.

Feel it continue traveling down your legs all the way down to your toes.

Your whole body is now filled with divine healing light and energy.

Allow that healing energy to completely fill any physical area that needs healing energy.

Feel it warming, healing and expanding through the area……creating space and relaxation.

Allow the healing light to bring peace and healing to any difficult emotions.

Bring your awareness to any intentions or desires that you may have.

Hold the thoughts of those intentions or desires as you allow the healing energy to manifest them for you.

Feel your connection to divine energy and light, and know that all is connected.

We are all connected, all is one.

Stay with this deep, relaxing, peaceful feeling of bliss as you navigate through the remainder of your day.

Take a few gentle breaths in and out.

Now, open your eyes slowly and give yourself a few moments to readjust to your physical surroundings.

When you are ready, roll on to your right side and push yourself back up to a seated position.

Before you leave class today, don't forget to thank yourself

for showing up on your mat today to nurture your mind, body, and spirit.

And thank you all so much for sharing this practice with me today.

Namaste.

12

Loving Kindness Meditation Script

Script and Guidance Tips:

- *Prepare the space for your students. Adjust the lighting, music, etc to create a calming and space environment*
- *Engage your students with a brief story, quote, or topic related to the following meditation to help shift their focus onto the practice*
- *On average, you should pause for 3 seconds between each line of the script*

—BEGIN READING HERE—

"Come to a comfortable position lying on your back.

Take a moment to get comfortable here and begin to focus on the natural rhythm of your breath.

Inhale slowly and smoothly allowing the breath to travel deeply into the low belly.

Pause and exhale slowly and smoothly releasing the breath from the body through your nostrils or out of your mouth."

- *Pause here for a few minutes in silence and let your students enter into a more relaxed and introspective space. Remind your students that your voice will be absent periodically throughout the practice. This is intentional - the silence allows them to turn their focus inward on their own journey through the practice.*
- *Remember to insert as many additional pauses as you need to. Your goal is to sound authentic and natural.*

"Now take a moment to make any last minute adjustments here so that your body can remain as comfortable and still as possible throughout this practice.

Feel the breath flowing in and flowing out.

Soften your face and jaw to allow the breath to flow smoothly in and smoothly out.

Soften the eyes and relax the shoulders.

Let your entire body feel relaxed and heavy.

Weighted and secure.

And now, slowly come back to the sound of my voice.

Keeping your eyes closed, think of a person close to you who loves you very much.

It could be someone from the past or the present; someone still in life or who has passed;

it could be a spiritual teacher or guide.

Imagine that person standing in front of you, sending you their love.

That person is sending you wishes for your safety, for your well being and happiness.

Feel the warm wishes and love coming from that person towards you.

Now imagine that you are surrounded on all sides by all the people who love you and have loved you.

Picture all of your friends and loved ones surrounding you.

They are standing sending you wishes for your happiness, well-being, and health.

Bask in the warm wishes and love coming from all sides.

You are filled, and overflowing with warmth and love.

Now picture a person that you love, perhaps a relative or a friend.

Begin to send the love that you feel back to that person.

You and this person are similar.

Just like you, this person wishes to be happy and have a good life.

Send all your love and warm wishes to that person.

Send all your wishes for well-being to that person, repeating the following phrase, silently: "Just as I wish to, may you live with ease, may you be happy, may you be safe and healthy"

Now think of an acquaintance, someone you don't know very well and toward whom you do not have any particular feeling.

It could be a neighbor, or a colleague, or someone else that you see around but do not know very well. You and this person are alike in your wish to have a good life.

Like you, this person wishes to experience joy and happiness in his or her life.

Send all your wishes for well-being to that person, repeating the following phrase, silently: "Just as I wish to, may you live with ease, may you be happy, may you be safe and healthy"

Now think of someone that you may not get along with. It may be someone that you have long-standing difficulties with.

Call the difficult person to mind, and be honest about what you feel.

There may well be feelings of discomfort.

Notice any tendency you may have to think badly of that person, or to deepen the conflict you have with them, and let go of these tendencies.

Instead, wish them well,repeating the following phrase, silently: "Just as I wish, may you live with ease, may you be happy, may you be safe and healthy"

Now expand your awareness and picture the whole globe in front of you as a little ball.

Send warm wishes to all living beings on the globe, who, like you, want to be happy: "Just as I wish to, may you live with ease, may you be happy, may you be safe and healthy"

Take a deep breath in. And breathe out.

And another deep breath in and let it go.

Notice the state of your mind and how you feel after this meditation.

Now, open your eyes slowly and give yourself a few moments to readjust to your physical surroundings.

When you are ready, roll on to your right side and push yourself back up to a seated position.

Before you leave class today, don't forget to thank yourself

for showing up on your mat today to nurture your mind, body, and spirit.

And thank you all so much for sharing this practice with me today.

Namaste.

13

Gratitude Meditation Script

Script and Guidance Tips:

- *Prepare the space for your students. Adjust the lighting, music, etc to create a calming and space environment*
- *Engage your students with a brief story, quote, or topic related to the following meditation to help shift their focus onto the practice*
- *On average, you should pause for 3 seconds between each line of the script*

—BEGIN READING HERE—

"Come to a comfortable position lying on your back.

Take a moment to get comfortable here and begin to focus on the natural rhythm of your breath.

Inhale slowly and smoothly allowing the breath to travel deeply into the low belly.

Pause and exhale slowly and smoothly releasing the breath from the body

through your nostrils or out of your mouth."

- *Pause here for a few minutes in silence and let your students enter into a more relaxed and introspective space. Remind your students that your voice will be absent periodically throughout the practice. This is intentional - the silence allows them to turn their focus inward on their own journey through the practice.*
- *Remember to insert as many additional pauses as you need to. Your goal is to sound authentic and natural.*

"Now take a moment to make any last minute adjustments here so that your body can remain as comfortable and still as possible throughout this practice.

Feel the breath flowing in and flowing out.

Soften your face and jaw to allow the breath to flow smoothly in and smoothly out.

Soften the eyes and relax the shoulders.

Let your entire body feel relaxed and heavy.

Weighted and secure.

And now, slowly come back to the sound of my voice.

Continue to breathe and let any distracting thoughts float away from you.

Feel gratitude for your family and your friends; for their love and support however it is given.

Feel gratitude for the community that surrounds and supports you.

Everyone from the grocer to your hair stylist, your dentist and doctor, your neighbors, co-workers, teachers and the person who serves you your favorite treat.

Let your heart expand to include your family, friends and community.

Gently breathe in and as you exhale allow your hips to soften and relax.

Rocking them back and forth, side to side to release any tension if that feels right today.

Feel gratitude for your creative mind. And for your dreams, desires and passions that allow you the ability to feel so very deeply.

Inhale feeling your belly expand, and exhale letting your belly relax and soften towards your spine.

Feel gratitude for the food that nourishes you and makes you strong.

Feel gratitude for your sense of self that defines who you are and allows you to serve the world in your special way.

Soften your ribs, your back and the area around your heart.

Feel your heart expand as you feel gratitude for the beauty of nature all around you. For the trees, plants and flowers, for the creatures that share our beautiful world.

Relax your shoulders, soften your arms from your shoulders all the way down to your fingertips.

Relax your jaw, your mouth, your tongue and your cheeks.

Feel gratitude for the gift of communication and all the ways you express yourself and share your story with the world.

Soften your eyes and your forehead. Allow the forehead to be free and clear.

Feel gratitude for your intuition; that little voice inside that guides you on the right path.

Feel gratitude for all the times you have listened and tuned into wisdom from within.

Soften the top of your head and sense the connection around you through your breath, feel connected to everything around you.

Feel gratitude for the connections that makes you whole and complete.

Enjoy this deep sense of peace that is now surrounding you.

Take a few gentle breaths in and out.

Now, open your eyes slowly and give yourself a few moments to readjust to your physical surroundings.

When you are ready, roll on to your right side and push yourself back up to a seated position.

Before you leave today, remember to feel gratitude for yourself.

For taking this time out of your day to meditate and take care of your mind body.

Thank you so much for sharing this practice with me today.

Namaste.

56

14

Forgiveness Meditation Script

Script and Guidance Tips:

- *Prepare the space for your students. Adjust the lighting, music, etc to create a calming and space environment*
- *Engage your students with a brief story, quote, or topic related to the following meditation to help shift their focus onto the practice*
- *On average, you should pause for 3 seconds between each line of the script*

—BEGIN READING HERE—

"Come to a comfortable position lying on your back.

Take a moment to get comfortable here and begin to focus on the natural rhythm of your breath.

Inhale slowly and smoothly allowing the breath to travel deeply into the low belly.

Pause and exhale slowly and smoothly releasing the breath from the body

through your nostrils or out of your mouth."

- *Pause here for a few minutes in silence and let your students enter into a more relaxed and introspective space. Remind your students that your voice will be absent periodically throughout the practice. This is intentional - the silence allows them to turn their focus inward on their own journey through the practice.*
- *Remember to insert as many additional pauses as you need to. Your goal is to sound authentic and natural.*

"Now take a moment to make any last minute adjustments here so that your body can remain as comfortable and still as possible throughout this practice.

Feel the breath flowing in and flowing out.

Soften your face and jaw to allow the breath to flow smoothly in and smoothly out.

Soften the eyes and relax the shoulders.

Let your entire body feel relaxed and heavy. Weighted and secure.

And now, slowly come back to the sound of my voice.

Continue to breathe and let any distracting thoughts float away from you.

Picture something that comes to mind that you judge yourself for.

Maybe you feel regret, or irritation, or sadness. Notice how it feels even bringing it to mind.

Then focus on these three phrases, not forcing anything but setting an intention:

I forgive myself for not understanding.

I forgive myself for making mistakes.

I forgive myself for causing pain and suffering to myself and others.

Bring your attention back again and focus on the three phrases:

I forgive myself for not understanding.

I forgive myself for making mistakes.

I forgive myself for causing pain and suffering to myself and others.

Now take a deep breath in through the nose.

And blow it out the mouth.

Allow yourself to settle and return when you're ready, now or maybe some time in the future.

Our mind naturally holds onto instances where we feel mistreated by others.

There may be experiences that were entirely wrong or traumatic or that concretely require our attention or action.

At the same time, we can practice avoiding the second arrow.

I forgive you for not understanding. I forgive you for making mistakes. I forgive you for causing pain and suffering to me and to others.

Letting go of the tendency to add resentment and judgment and everything related to challenging and unpleasant situations.

Again, if it's too much to consider, return to breathing, or if you prefer, focusing on compassion for yourself instead.

Practices of this kind can be quite challenging, so in these last few moments, on each in breath, noticing and accepting whatever you feel right now.

On each out-breath, as you would for a close friend, offering yourself relief, or freedom, or strength, or whatever first comes to mind.

Forgiveness doesn't mean being passive or not taking action. It doesn't mean standing down when we need to protect ourselves or someone else from harm.

Do what needs to be done— that might mean taking a pause, settling the mind, and trying to see things as clearly as possible before taking skillful action.

Continue to practice forgiveness, over and over again, letting go of whatever holds you back and know that

You are incredibly strong, you are incredibly brave.

You are safe here.

You are healing now

and above all else, you are loved.

Take a few gentle breaths in and out.

Now, open your eyes slowly and give yourself a few moments to readjust to your physical surroundings.

When you are ready, roll on to your right side and push yourself back up to a seated position.

Before you leave class today, don't forget to thank yourself

for showing up on your mat today to nurture your mind, body, and spirit.

And thank you all so much for sharing this practice with me today.

Namaste.

15

Yoga Nidra Script

Yoga Nidra "Yogic Sleep" Script:

Come down to lying on your mat in savasana. Take a few moments to make yourself as comfortable as possible. I recommend using props to support your body and maybe even a blanket to keep you warm throughout this practice of yoga nidra, or "yogic sleep". We will journey to a place between sleep and wakefulness. Listen to my voice to stay awake. You might affirm to yourself now, "I am practicing yoga nidra. I will stay awake." You will be guided on a journey of awareness moving from sensations to emotions and images. Focus only enough to stay awake. You don't need to worry about catching every detail.

Before we begin, take a moment to set an intention or "sankalpa" for your practice. Your intention should be in the present tense and begin with "I am". For example, you could say "I am at peace" or "I am loved". Choose your own sankalpa now and once you've decided on it close your eyes and recite it to yourself internally three times.

As you settle into Savasana, bring your awareness to the ground beneath you. Allow your body to soften and rest. As you settle into stillness, invite your body to melt into your mat.

Sense your whole body on the floor. Your whole body on the floor in this room. Here and now. Your whole body on the floor in this room.

We will begin a rotation of awareness. All you need to do is follow my voice as I guide you from point to point along your body.

Move your awareness to your mouth. Become aware of your tongue. Lower jaw. Lower row of teeth. Upper row of teeth. Gums. Upper lip. Lower lip. Space between your lips. Both cheeks. Right ear. Left ear. Forehead. Both temples. Top of the head. Back of the head. Tip of the nose. Right nostril. Left nostril. Right eyelid. Left eyelid. Right eye. Left eye. Right eyebrow. Left eyebrow. Space between the eyebrows. Now go to the right hand. The right hand thumb. Second finger. Third finger. Fourth finger. Little finger. Palm of the hand. Back of the hand. Wrist. Forearm. Elbow. Upper arm. Shoulder. Right armpit. Ribs. Waist. Hip. Right thigh. Knee. Calf. Ankle. Heel. Sole of the foot. Top of the foot. Right big toe. Second toe. Third toe. Fourth toe. Pinky toe. Go to the left hand. The left hand thumb. Second finger. Third finger. Fourth finger. Little finger. Palm of the hand. Back of the hand. Wrist. Forearm. Elbow. Upper arm. Shoulder. Left armpit. Ribs. Waist. Hip. Left thigh. Knee. Calf. Ankle. Heel. Sole of the foot. Top of the foot. Left big toe. Second toe. Third toe. Fourth toe. Pinky toe. Pelvis. Sit Bones. Lower back. Mid-back. Upper back. Right shoulder blade. Left shoulder blade. Back of the neck. Back of the head. Right inner ear. Left inner ear. Roof of the mouth. Throat. Right collar bone. Left collar bone. Right chest. Left chest. Middle chest. Upper abdomen. Navel. Lower abdomen. Pelvis. Whole spine. The whole head. Right arm. Left arm. Both arms together. The whole right leg. The whole left leg. Both legs together. Whole front body. Whole back body.

Become aware of the whole body.

Now bring your awareness to your breath. Follow the gentle tide of your breath without altering it. Now, picture your breath as a bright white light swirling up and down your spinal column. On your next inhale, this light travels from the tailbone to the top of the head. As you exhale, it moves from the crown of the head back down to the tailbone. the golden light flows from the tailbone to the crown of the head. Stay with your breath as it flows up and down your spinal column, delivering fresh oxygen and loosening any existing tension between the vertebrae.

Now imagine your body is very heavy. Feel the earth pulling you down. You are feeling so grounded. Head heavy. Arms and legs heavy. Torso heavy. Sinking down…

Now Imagine your body is so light you could float up and away. Head light, torso light, arms and legs …weightless. Gently flutter back down like a feather. Reconnecting with the earth beneath you.

Feel your lips and jaw and relax. Feel the back of your head on the floor, relaxed. Feel the space between your eyebrows, relaxed.

Now visualize the following things for a few moments each, allowing them to pass through your mind as if they were on a roll of film.

The color blue
Looking out the window on a rainy day.
A mother smiling.
The sun shining.
You, laughing.
And the color green.

Just feel yourself and let yourself be held by the earth. In the most nourishing ocean, floating effortlessly. Everything is loose, limber. At peace. Your whole body, relaxed.

Now repeat your sankalpa 3 times, quietly, internally and with meaning.

[PAUSE FOR FIVE MINUTES]

The practice of yoga nidra is now complete.

Gently draw your awareness back into your physical body. Start to wiggle your toes and fingers. Become aware of your breath. Without opening your eyes, become aware of your surroundings. Take all the time you need….but when you feel ready, slowly roll over onto your right side. Take several moments here. Just breathe.

Then when you're ready, gently press up to a comfortable seat.

And thank you all so much for sharing this practice with me today.

Namaste.

16

Object Focused Candle Meditation Script

Script and Guidance Tips:

- *Prepare the space for your students. Adjust the lighting, music, etc to create a calming and space environment*
- *Engage your students with a brief story, quote, or topic related to the following meditation to help shift their focus onto the practice*
- *On average, you should pause for 3 seconds between each line of the script*

Preparing the Space for Candle Meditations:

Give each of your students a tea light placed on a non-flammable plate. Place the light on top of a sturdy surface like a yoga block or a stack of solid books. Place the pedestal with the candle on it up against the wall. Have your students seated facing the wall about 2-3 feet from the candle with their gaze directed at the candle. Yoga mats should be placed with the short end against the wall for this exercise. Bolsters and meditation cushions work perfectly fine too.

—BEGIN READING HERE—

To begin our candle meditation, bring yourself to a seated position.

Take note of how your body feels.

Take a deep breath in, and as you exhale, notice where your body feels the most tense.

Focus on these areas as you take another breath.

Allow the tension to flow away as you breathe out.

Inhale as you raise your shoulders… then relax as you exhale, and lower your shoulders into a comfortable position.

Continue to breathe smoothly and gently as you go forward through this meditation.

Rest peacefully in your easy seated position, maintaining a straight but comfortable spine.

Begin to settle into your surroundings as I come around and light each of your candles.

The room is pleasantly dark, and you are safe and comfortable.

Close your eyes for a minute or two and begin to focus on and deepen the breath.

Now open your eyes.

Look directly at the candle flame in front of you.

Observe the glow of a candle.

Keep your attention facing forward as you notice the gentle flickers of warm light on the wall in front of you.

See the dancing light from the candle.

Feel yourself relaxing as you watch the beautiful patterns made by the light of the candle.

Continue to observe the candle and stay here in this moment for a few minutes.

Acknowledging only your breath and the candle in front of you.

Now close your eyes and keep them closed for the next few minutes.

Picture the candle in front of you, and see the soft light it creates.

Notice the flame gently moving as the candle burns.

Imagine what the candle looks like.

What shape is it? What color? What size?

Create a picture of the candle in your mind.

Imagine that the candle gently melts away the stresses and tension you have been holding in your body.

As the candle burns, feel the tension easing, and relaxation flowing through your body.

Imagine the wax becoming softer.

Feel your body also becoming softer.

The softening wax is melting, turning to liquid.

Warm and flowing.…. free from tension.…..

Open your eyes again and view the soft flame at the top of the candle.

See how it flickers slightly in response to your breath as you exhale.

Watch how the flame responds each time you breathe.

See the wax of the candle melting.…melting the way your tension is melting away.

It feels like any stresses you were holding on to are dripping away with each drop of wax from the candle.

The soft flame of relaxation warms you from the inside, melting away all stress.

Watch the wax melting.…. feeling the same effects on the tension in your body.

Melting.…. relaxing.

Continue to observe the burning candle, enjoying the relaxation you are experiencing.

When you are ready to finish your relaxation session, take a deep breath.…. and exhale through your mouth, blowing out the candle.

Slowly bring your awareness back to the present.

Become more aware of the time and place you are in today

Enjoy the feeling of calm and peace that remains with you.

Namaste.

17

Namaste, Friends!

Deepest thanks to my compassionate, creative, and forward-thinking readers. Never doubt that you were put on this earth to embrace others with your warmth and wisdom.

Guided Meditation Scripts: A Teaching Resource for Yoga Instructors, Life Coaches, Wellness Gurus and Healers

Revised 2nd Edition August 2022

Written By: Sandra L. Knecht